Herbal Home Remedies for Gingival (Gum) Diseases: A Hand Book

Authors

Dr. P.L Ravishankar, MDS
Professor & Head, Department of Periodontics, SRM Kattankulathur Dental College & Hospital, Potheri, Tamil Nadu, India

Dr. Shatabdy Das, BDS
Kumudini Medical College and Hospital, Dhaka, Bangladesh

Dr. Maharshi Malakar, MDS
Department of Periodontics, SRM Kattankulathur Dental College & Hospital, Potheri, Kattankulathur, Tamil Nadu, India

AkiNik Publications
New Delhi

Published By: *AkiNik Publications*

AkiNik Publications
169, C-11, Sector - 3,
Rohini, Delhi-110085, India
Toll Free (India) – 18001234070

Author: *Dr. P.L Ravishankar, Dr. Shatabdy Das and Dr. Maharshi Malakar.*

1st Edition: *2018*

Pages: *23*

ISBN: *978-93-88112-67-3*

Price: *₹235/-*

Contents

Chapter - 1

Introduction

Gingiva (Gum) is pinkish coloured soft tissue holding the teeth in bony sockets by adhering them firmly through periodontal ligaments to periosteum. It is the major cause of tooth loss in later half of life as in adult as well as in elderly. In early stages it is called gingivitis and when gingivitis is not treated properly, it may advance to periodontitis because of nonspecific signs and symptoms to be noted by patients. Main reasons for gum diseases are following-

- Non-specific symptoms
- Economical
- Educational
- psycho-social
- ignorance
- self-medication
- Economical factors

Dental treatments and dental care is supposed to be costlier affair in a dental clinic as compared to medical services in general. In government sector dental facilities are less as compared to load of population as well as shortage of dental clinics in government sector.

Factors Which Increases/Causes Gum Disease-

- Poor oral hygiene
- Smoking or Chewing tobacco
- Genetic
- Patient having chronic medical condition like diabetes, epilepsy, leukemia etc.
- Person taking high physical and emotional stresses.
- Occur by hormonal changes like pregnancy, puberty, menopause etc.
- Vitamin C deficiency

- Faulty dentistry
- Mouth breather
- Toothbrush trauma
- Clenching and grinding of teeth

Medication includes steroids and certain types of anti-epileptic drugs, cancer therapy, calcium channel blockers and oral contraceptives.

Warning sign that can signal gum problems:

- Gum that bleed easily
- Red, swollen, tender gums
- Gum that have pulled from the teeth
- Permanent teeth that are loose or separating
- Any change in the way your teeth fit together when you bite

Chapter - 2

Gingivitis

Gingivitis means inflammation of the gums, or gingiva. It commonly occurs because a film of plaque, or bacteria, accumulates on the teeth.

Gingivitis is a non-destructive type of periodontal disease, but untreated gingivitis can progress to periodontitis. This is more serious and can eventually lead to loss of teeth.

Signs of gingivitis include red and puffy gums that bleed easily when the person brushes their teeth. Gingivitis often resolves with good oral hygiene, such as longer and more frequent brushing, and flossing. In addition, an antiseptic mouthwash may help.

In mild cases of gingivitis, patients may not even know they have it, because symptoms are mild. However, the condition should be taken seriously and addressed immediately.

Types

There are two main categories of gingival diseases:

Dental plaque-induced gingival disease: This can be caused by plaque, systemic factors, medications, or malnutrition.

Non-plaque induced gingival lesions: This can be caused by a specific bacterium, virus, or fungus. It might also be caused by genetic factors, systemic conditions (including allergic reactions and certain illnesses), wounds, or reactions to foreign bodies, such as dentures. Sometimes, there is no specific cause.

Causes

The most common cause of gingivitis is the accumulation of bacterial plaque between and around the teeth. The plaque triggers an immune response, which, in turn, can eventually lead to the destruction of gingival, or gum, tissue. It may also, eventually, lead to further complications, including the loss of teeth.

Dental Plaque

Dental plaque is a biofilm that accumulates naturally on the teeth. It is usually formed by colonizing bacteria that are trying to stick to the smooth surface of a tooth.

These bacteria might help protect the mouth from the colonization of harmful microorganisms, but dental plaque can also cause tooth decay, and periodontal problems such as gingivitis and chronic periodontitis, a gum infection.

When plaque is not removed adequately, it can harden into calculus, or tartar, at the base of the teeth, near the gums. This has a yellow color. Calculus can only be removed professionally.

Plaque and tartar eventually irritate the gums, causing gum inflammation around the base of the teeth. This means that the gums might easily bleed.

Poor Oral Hygiene

Poor oral hygiene, such as not brushing teeth properly or regularly can cause plaque to build up in your teeth. If plaque is not removed it can harden form a substance called tartar [calculus]. Tartar sticks much firmly on the teeth than plaque and usually only be removed by dentists. The non-mineralised plaque on calculus surface is principal irritants but the underlying calcified portion may be a significant contributing factor. It does not irritate the gingival directly, but it provides a fixed nisus for the continued accumulation of the irritating surface plaque and holds the plaque against gingival. Calculus is a significant pathogenic factor in periodontal disease. Bacteria in plaque will irritate gums, making them inflamed and sore. If gum disease is not treated and plaque and tartar continues to build which develops periodontal can cause teeth loose and eventually falling out.

Smoking and Chewing Tobacco

Smoking and chewing tobacco is a risk factor for gum disease because chemical inhaled interfere with the body's ability to repair damaged tissue. Smoking cut down on the blood supply because it is vasoconstrictive. It limits the flow of oxygen and nutrients to the tissue. It is also known that nicotine is toxic to the cells called fibroblasts which are responsible for manufacture new connective tissue. The less fibroblast work, the more rapid progression of gum disease.

Genetic

Genetic factor may play the critical role in half the cases of periodontal disease. Up to 30% of the population may have some genetic susceptibility to periodontal disease. Some people with severe periodontal disease have genetic factor that effect. The immune factor interleukin-1, a cytokine involved in the inflammatory response. Such individual are up to 20 times more likely to develop advanced Periodontitis than those without these genetic factor.

Person Having Systemic Conditions

Diabetes: It is estimated that 1 in 3 diabetic suffer from Periodontitis at some stage of their diseases. When diabetes is poorly managed it can lead to Periodontitis in both children and adults. When a body is suffering from diabetes, the structure of the blood vessels is altered. This may affect the efficiency of blood flow, and in turn may weaken the bone and the gums leaving them more prone to infection. Furthermore, if diabetes is not strictly managed, there may be higher than usual level of glucose in the mouth fluid which encourages the growth of gum disease- causing bacteria.

HIV: HIV gingivitis is also called linear gingival erythema, brightly inflamed marginal gingivitis gingival can be painful and bleed easily and there may be rapid tissue destruction. In HIV gingivitis organism are primarily gram negative anaerobes, enteric strains and yeast that are not found in routine cases of gingivitis. Treatment consists of debridement plus antibiotic administration. Antifungal rinses as well as Antibacterial rinses are also required.

Leukemia: Particularly the monotypic type can cause gingival enlargement due to infiltration of gingival tissue. Gingival enlargement due to leukaemia is typically oedematous and haemorrhagic. Patient with gingival hypertrophy have difficulty in maintaining good oral hygiene due to gingival bleeding.

Person taking high physical and emotional stresses- Stress elevates the level of stress hormone cortical which affect the gums. Stress may make people more lax about their oral health. Individual with high stress level tend to increase their bad habits like use of nicotine, alcohol or drugs which can be harmful to periodontal health.

Other Causes and Risk Factors

Changes in Hormones: This may occur during puberty, menopause, the menstrual cycle, and pregnancy. The gingiva might become more sensitive, raising the risk of inflammation.

Drugs: Oral health may be affected by some medications, especially if saliva flow is reduced. Dilantin, an anticonvulsant, and some anti-angina medications can cause abnormal growth of gum tissue.

Smoking: Regular smokers more commonly develop gingivitis, compared with non-smokers.

Age: The risk of gingivitis increases with age.

Poor Diet: A vitamin-C deficiency, for example, is linked to gum disease.

Family History: Those whose parent or parents have had gingivitis have a higher risk of developing it too. This is thought to be due to the type of bacteria we acquire during our early life.

Mouth ulcers are painful areas in the mouth and gums, they are also known as canker sores.

Signs and Symptoms

In mild cases of gingivitis, there may be no discomfort or noticeable symptoms.

Signs and symptoms of gingivitis might include: The symptoms of gingivitis are somewhat non-specific and manifest in the gum tissue as the classic signs of inflammation:

Swollen gums

Bright red or purple gumstender gums that may be painful to the touch

Bleeding from the gums when brushing or flossing

Halitosis, or bad breath

Inflammation, or swollen gums

Receding gums

Soft gums

Gums that are tender or painful to the touch

Bleeding gums or bleeding after brushing and/or flossing

Bad breath (halitosis)

Additionally, the stippling that normally exists in the gum tissue of some individuals will often disappear and the gums may appear shiny when the gum tissue becomes swollen and stretched over the inflamed underlying connective tissue. The accumulation may also emit an unpleasant odor. When the gingiva are swollen, the epithelial lining of the gingival crevice becomes ulcerated and the gums will bleed more easily with even gentle brushing, and especially when flossing.

Complications

Recurrence of gingivitis

Periodontitis

Infection or abscess of the gingiva or the jaw bones

Trench mouth (bacterial infection and ulceration of the gums)

Swollen lymph nodes

Associated with premature birth and low birth weight [5]

Diagnosis

A dentist or oral hygienist will check for symptoms, such as plaque and tartar in the oral cavity.

Checking for signs of periodontitis may also be recommended. This may be done by X-ray or periodontal probing, using an instrument that measures pocket depths around a tooth.

Treatment

If diagnosis happens early, and if treatment is prompt and proper, gingivitis can be successfully reversed.

Treatment involves care by a dental professional, and follow-up procedures carried out by the patient at home.

Professional dental care

Teeth before and after scaling

Teeth before scaling and 9 days after.

Plaque and tartar are removed. This is known as scaling. This can be uncomfortable, especially if tartar build-up is extensive, or the gums are very sensitive.

The dental professional will explain the importance of oral hygiene and how to brush and floss effectively.

Follow-up appointments may be recommended, with more frequent cleanings if necessary.

Fixing any damaged teeth also contributes to oral hygiene.

Chapter - 3

Home Remedies for Gum Disease

The simplest and most common way to relieve pain and discomfort from gum disease is to rinse your mouth with warm water mixed with some salt.

Here are 10 home remedies for gum disease:-

1. Hydrogen Peroxide

Hydrogen peroxide works as a strong antibacterial agent that kills germs and fights gum disease. Plus, it helps whiten and brighten your pearly whites. Make sure you use the 3 percent hydrogen peroxide solution that typically comes in brown bottles, rather than the highly concentrated version.

Mix equal parts of hydrogen peroxide and water. Rinse your mouth with the solution for a few seconds, and then spit it out. Use it a few times a week until you are satisfied with the results.

Alternatively, mix hydrogen peroxide little by little into one teaspoon of baking soda to make a paste. Put the paste on your toothbrush and gently brush it on your gums and gum line. Finally, spit it out and rinse your mouth. Use it a few times a week for a few weeks.

You can also apply a paste of clove oil and hydrogen peroxide, leave it on for a few seconds and then spit it out. Repeat as needed.

Note: Do not use hydrogen peroxide too often; once a day is sufficient. Do not swallow it.

2. Aloe Vera

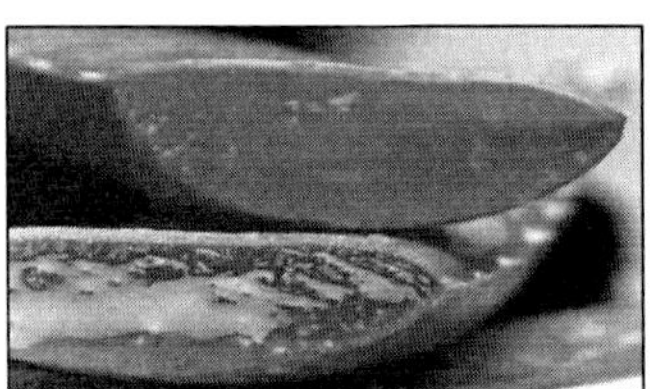

Due to its anti-inflammatory and healing properties, aloe vera has been found to be beneficial in dealing with gum disease. Being an antimicrobial, it also kills the bacteria that cause gum disease. Plus, it fights bad breath and heals mouth ulcers.

Massage your gums with fresh aloe vera gel, leave it on for at least half an hour and then rinse it off. Repeat several times a day.

Alternatively, swish some aloe vera juice around in your mouth a few times, and then spit it out.

You can also drink about two teaspoons of aloe vera juice on a regular basis.

Follow any of these remedies daily for several weeks.

Note: Drinking too much aloe vera juice can have a laxative effect.

3. Cranberry Juice

Cranberry juice is good for fighting gum disease and infection due to its high vitamin C content. A study published in the Journal of Periodontology has associated lower intake of vitamin C with higher rates of periodontal disease.

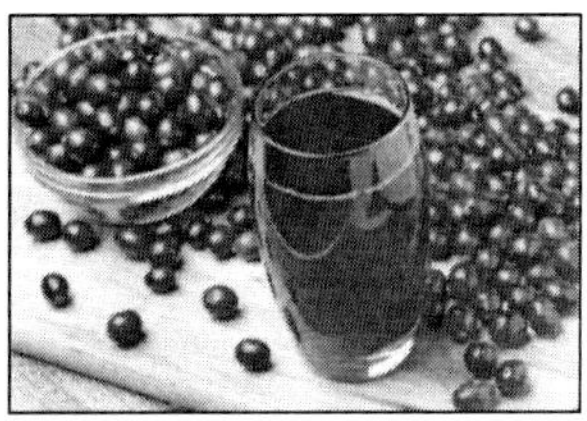

Simply drink about four ounces, or two tablespoons, of cranberry juice daily to help prevent bacteria from sticking to your teeth.

Plus, eat more vitamin C-rich fruits and vegetables, such as lemons, oranges, grapefruits, blueberries, strawberries, papaya, red pepper and broccoli.

4. Oil Pulling

Oil pulling is a traditional Ayurvedic technique that is excellent for oral care. It helps strengthen the teeth and gums, reduces plaque, and relieves bad breath. It is also considered good for overall health as it removes toxins.

Swish one tablespoon of sesame oil around in your mouth and through your teeth.

Do this for about 15 minutes or until it becomes thinner and turns milky.

Spit it out and rinse your mouth with water.

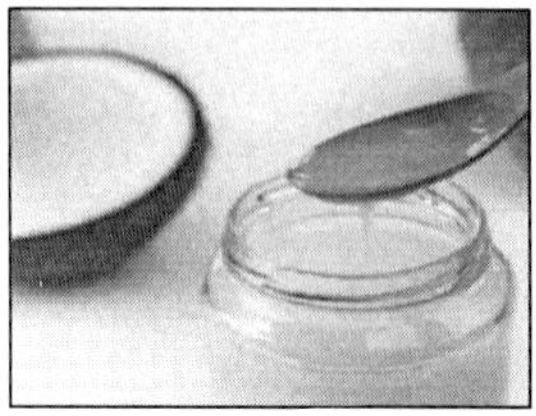

Repeat the process daily for about a month.

For better results, use coconut oil for oil pulling.

Note: Do not gargle or swallow the oil.

5. Myrrh

Myrrh is good for treating gum disease and maintaining proper oral hygiene because it has antiseptic, antibacterial and astringent properties. It is often recommended by herbalists as a remedy for sore gums.

Put 10 drops of myrrh tincture in a cup of warm water and use it as a mouth rinse. You can also add a few drops of the tincture to a salt water rinse. Repeat once or twice a day for several days.

Alternatively, mix equal amounts of myrrh and Echinacea tinctures. Use this as a mouth rinse. Repeat daily for a few days until you get relief.

6. Tea Tree Oil

The anti-inflammatory properties of tea tree oil help soothe irritated and inflamed gums. A study published in the Australian Dental Journal in 2008 found that topical application of a tea tree oil gel helped reduce gum bleeding and gingivitis. It did not reduce plaque though.

Simply put a few drops of tea tree oil

7. Sea Salt

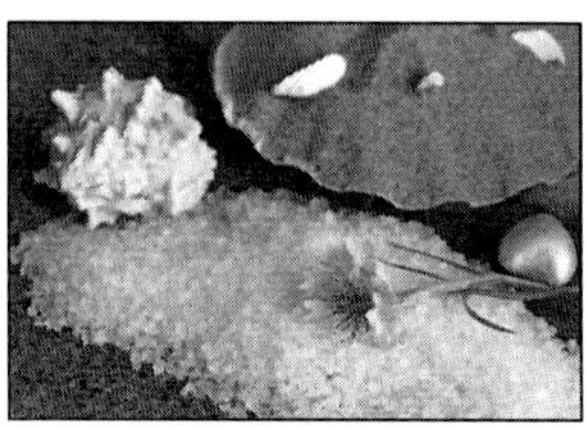

Natural sea salt contains minerals that reduce inflammation, ease pain and draw out any infection.

Mix a small amount of sea salt in a cup of warm water until it dissolves completely.

Use it as a mouth rinse, swishing it around in your mouth for a few seconds.

Do this three times a day until your symptoms subside.

8. Tea Bags

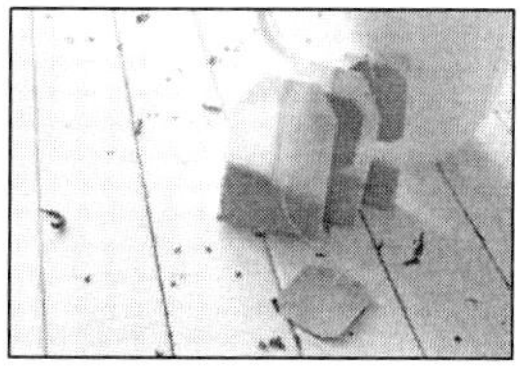

Tea, particularly black tea, contains tannic acid that helps reduce pain and inflammation. In addition, it contains antioxidants that help fight infections.

Steep a tea bag in hot water for 10 minutes, and then allow it to cool.

Place the tea bag on the affected area for three to five minutes.

Repeat a few times a day until you get relief.

9. Coconut Oil

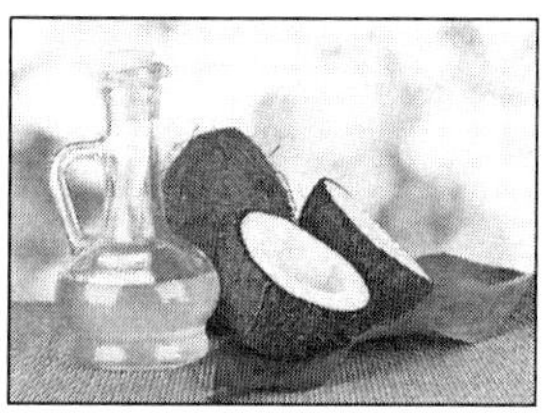

The antibacterial and anti-inflammatory properties of coconut oil help in the natural treatment of gum disease. Combining it with baking soda will help neutralize the acids in your mouth, too.

1. Mix two tablespoons each of coconut oil and baking soda.
2. Use this in place of your toothpaste once or twice a week on a regular basis.

10. Chamomile Tea

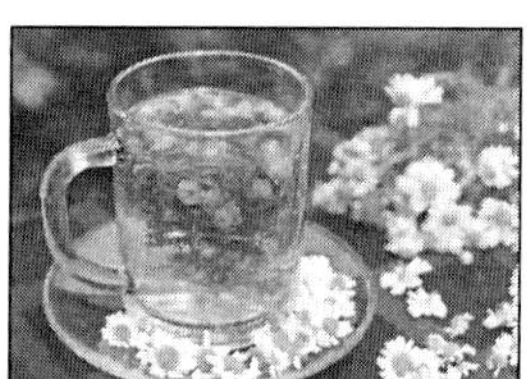

Chamomile tea helps ease pain and inflammation associated with gum disease due to its anti-inflammatory and antiseptic properties.

1. Add two to three teaspoons of chamomile flowers to one cup of hot water.
2. Let it steep for 10 minutes.
3. Strain and let it cool.
4. Use this chamomile tea as a mouth rinse a few times a day until you notice improvement.

In addition to these remedies, make sure to maintain adequate oral hygiene, including daily brushing, flossing and using a mouth rinse to reduce plaque buildup on your teeth. Plus, get regular dental check-ups.

Chapter - 4

Home Remedies for Periodontitis (Pyorrhea)

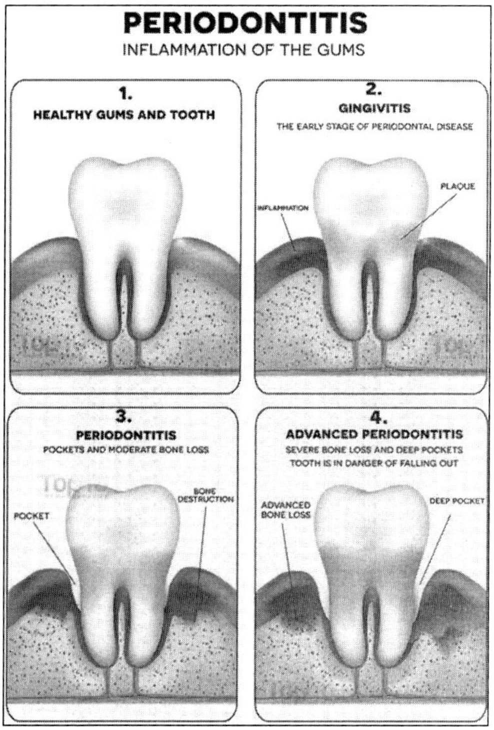

Note: Do consult a dentist for proper diagnosis and treatment of this condition. Use home remedies just as an adjunct treatment.

Periodontitis, formerly known as pyorrhea, is an advanced stage of gum disease in which the gums and bones that provide support to the teeth become inflamed and infected.

It usually happens due to advanced gingivitis, which when left untreated results in long-term accumulation of bacterial plaque and tartar on the teeth.

The onset of periodontitis is marked by bleeding of the gums. Other common signs and symptoms are bad breath, inflamed or swollen gums, mouth ulcers, formation of deep pockets between the teeth and gums, pus between your teeth and gums, and loose teeth.

There are several factors that can put you at a higher risk of developing periodontitis.

They include gingivitis, heredity, excessive use of tobacco products, poor oral hygiene, age, diabetes, hormonal changes in the body during pregnancy or menopause, and using poor-fitting dental restorations.

If not treated timely, periodontitis can lead to loss of teeth. It can even increase the risk of heart attacks, strokes and other serious health problems.

Periodontitis is a common dental issue but largely preventable. It can be prevented by following a proper oral hygiene.

You can also use some simple home remedies for periodontitis. Plus, proper treatment by a qualified dentist is a must.

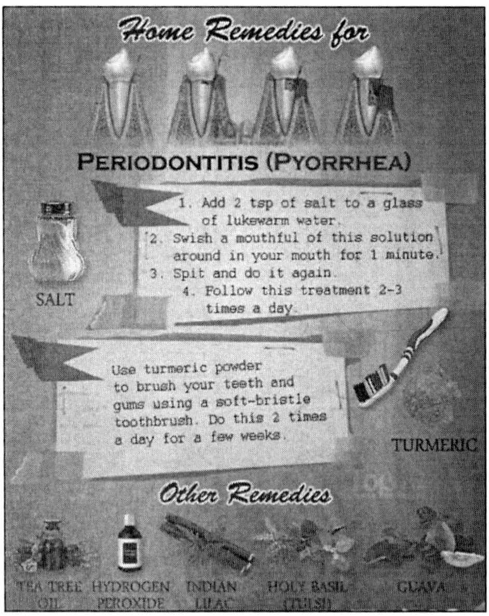

Here are the 10 home remedies for periodontitis.

1. Salt

The antiseptic and antibacterial properties of salt can take care of the bacteria that causes periodontitis. Plus, it can reduce inflammation and pain.

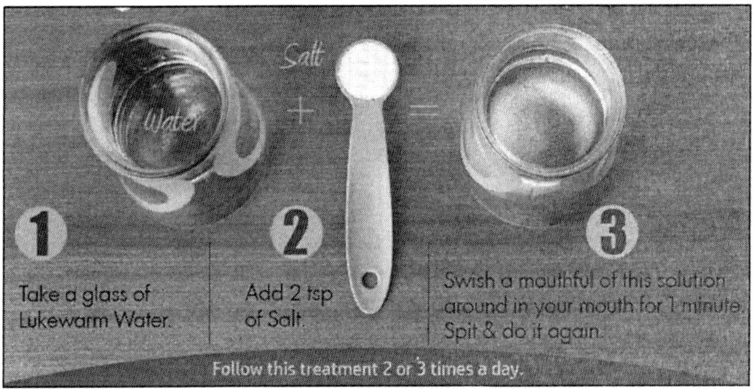

1. Add 2 teaspoons of salt to a glass of lukewarm water. Swish a mouthful of this solution around in your mouth for 1 minute. Spit and do it again. Follow this treatment 2 or 3 times a day.
2. Another option is to mix a pinch of salt and a little mustard oil to make a paste. After brushing your teeth, rub this mixture on the gums and leave it on for 5 minutes. Then, rinse thoroughly with warm water. Follow this remedy daily in the morning.

Use these remedies daily until your symptoms subside.

2. Oil Pulling

According to Ayurveda, oil pulling and gum massage can help prevent periodontitis and plaque buildup by reducing the amount of bacteria present in the mouth.

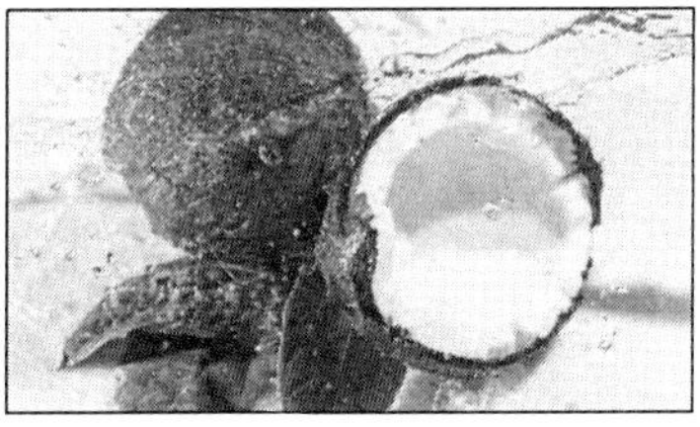

Oil pulling can even strengthen gums and promote good oral health. This has been proven by a study done in 2014 at Manipal College of Dental Sciences in India.

3. Swish a mouthful of organic, unrefined coconut oil or sesame oil around in your mouth for 15 to 20 minutes.
4. Spit it out and rinse your mouth with warm water.
5. Do this daily in the morning before brushing your teeth.

Note: Do not gargle or swallow the oil.

3. Turmeric

Turmeric contains curcumin, which has antibacterial and anti-inflammatory effects.

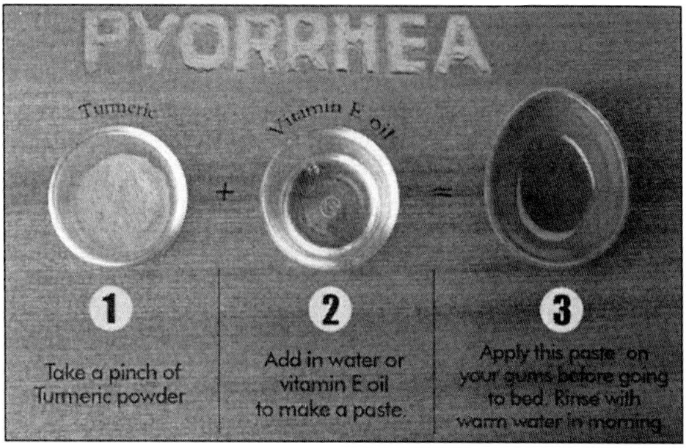

Turmeric can easily kill the bacteria present in the gums as well as relieve pain and inflammation. It also promotes oral health.

1. Use turmeric powder to brush your teeth and gums using a soft-bristle toothbrush. Do this 2 times a day for a few weeks.
2. Alternatively, prepare a gum pack with turmeric to treat periodontitis. Mix a pinch of turmeric powder with a little water or vitamin E oil to make a paste. Apply it on your gums before going to bed. The next morning, rinse your mouth with warm water. Do this once daily for several weeks.

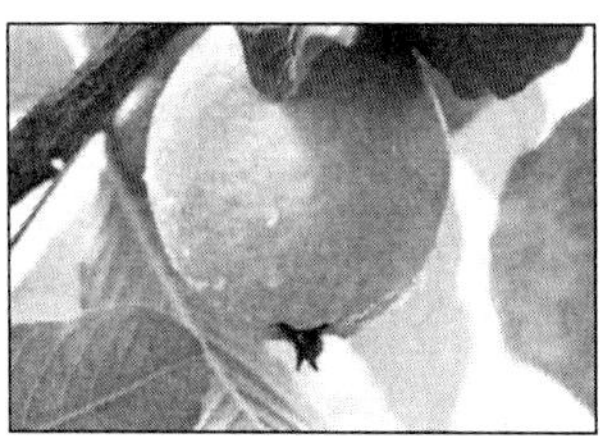

4. Guava

Being rich in vitamin C, guava is also considered an excellent remedy for periodontitis. It works as an anti-plaque agent and helps remove plaque accumulated on the teeth and gums. Plus, its anti-inflammatory and analgesic properties help reduce swelling and pain on the gums.

1. Wash some tender guava leaves. Chew the leaves thoroughly, then spit them out. Do this on a regular basis to stop bleeding and reduce the risk of pus forming in the gums.

2. Another option is to cut an unripe guava into four pieces. Sprinkle salt on the guava pieces and chew them slowly. It will help reduce plaque and make your gums and teeth strong.

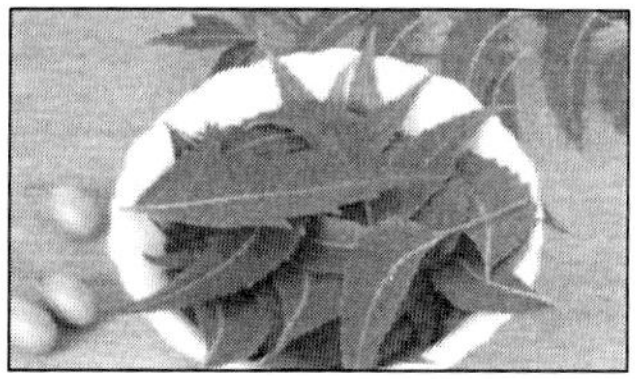

5. Indian Lilac

Indian lilac, also known as neem, is also very beneficial in getting rid of periodontitis. Its antibacterial properties help keep your gums free from harmful bacteria. Plus, it helps combat bad breath and keeps your gums and teeth healthy.

1. Extract the juice from a few neem leaves. Apply this juice on the gums and teeth, allow it to sit for 5 minutes and then rinse it off with warm water. Follow this treatment 1 or 2 times daily.

2. You can also use soft neem twigs to brush your teeth and gums twice daily.

6. Hydrogen Peroxide

Hydrogen peroxide has antibacterial properties that help kill germs and fight gum disease.

Additionally, it will help whiten your teeth. It is recommended to use food grade, 3 percent hydrogen peroxide solution only.

1. Prepare a solution with equal parts of hydrogen peroxide and water. Use it to rinse your mouth for a few seconds, and then spit it out.

2. Another option is to mix 1 teaspoon of baking soda and enough hydrogen peroxide to make a paste. With your fingers, rub your gums and gum line with this paste. Spit it out and rinse your mouth thoroughly.

Follow either treatment only 2 or 3 times a week until you get the desired result. Do not use hydrogen peroxide daily.

7. Holy Basil

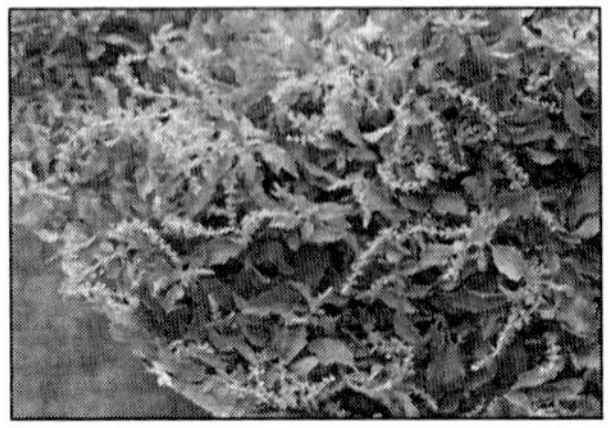

Holy basil is a good remedy for treating bleeding gums, one of the most common symptoms of periodontitis. Its antibacterial property can reduce the effect of harmful bacteria in the mouth. It also helps safeguard against other dental problems like toothaches and pus or pain in the gums.

- Mix 1 teaspoon of dried and powdered holy basil leaves with enough mustard oil to make a paste. Rub this paste on your teeth and gums and brush gently using a soft-bristle toothbrush. Do this 2 times a day for several weeks.
- You can also drink a few cups of basil tea daily or use it to rinse your mouth to treat and prevent periodontitis.

8. Cayenne Pepper

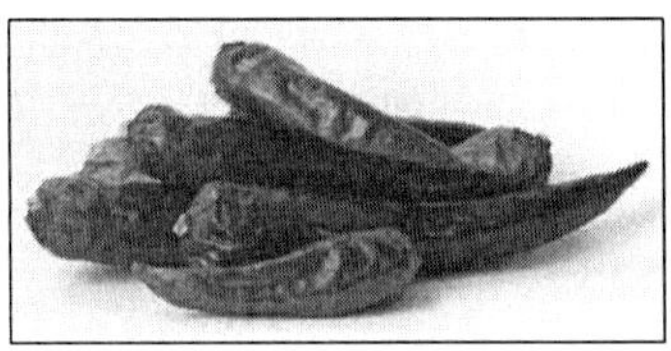

Cayenne pepper has anti-inflammatory properties that can help reduce swelling of the gums caused by periodontitis. Being rich in capsaicin, cayenne pepper also helps reduce pain.

1. Put a few drops of cayenne pepper tincture on a soft-bristle toothbrush.
2. Use it to brush your gums for a few minutes.
3. Rinse your mouth thoroughly with water.
4. Follow this treatment once daily to help relieve pain and reverse periodontitis.

Note: You can do oil pulling after using this remedy to reduce the stinging or burning sensation

9. **Tea Tree Oil**

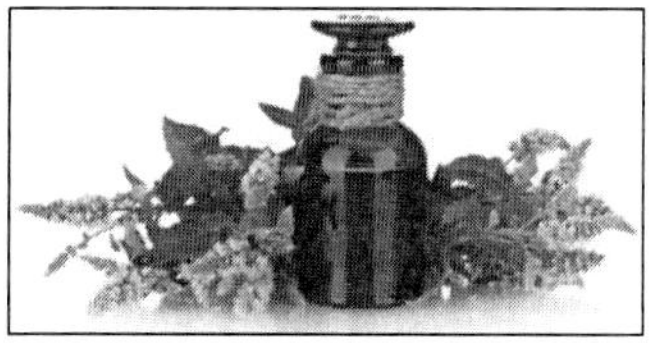

Tea tree oil has natural antibacterial and antiseptic properties that help fight microorganisms. Plus, it helps reduce bleeding and gingival inflammation. Tea tree oil is also beneficial for other dental issues like oral thrush and herpes.

- Apply tea tree oil in the form of gel using a toothbrush, twice daily for several weeks.
- Another option is to add a drop of tea tree in your regular toothpaste and brush your teeth with it, twice daily.

Note: Do not swallow tea tree oil.

10. **Black Pepper**

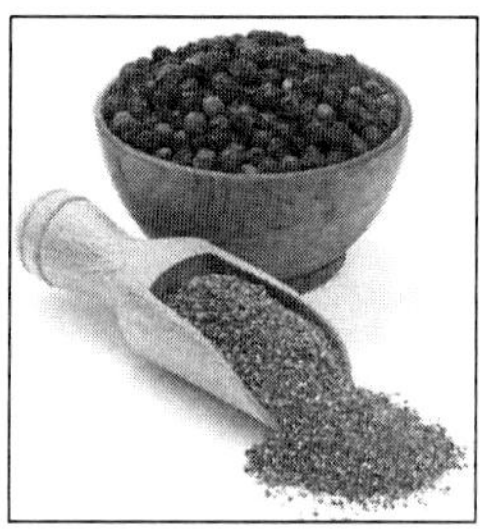

According to Ayurveda, black pepper is another excellent remedy for periodontitis. Its medicinal properties help reduce bacterial infection by getting rid of plaque and tartar on the teeth and gums. Also, it helps strengthen the gums.

- One simple option is to prepare a mixture of equal amounts of finely powdered black pepper and salt. Use it to massage the gums gently 2 or 3 times a day.
- Another option is to prepare a mixture of 2 teaspoons of crushed pomegranate seeds, ½ teaspoon of pepper powder and 1 teaspoon of salt. Apply it on the gums. Massage for 2 to 3 minutes, then rinse with

- Warm water. Do this once daily.

Tea Bags

Put a tea bag in the boiling water. Remove it and let it cool. Once cooled, place the tea bag on the infected part of the gum. Hold it there for approximately 5 minutes. You will definitely feel comfortable. The tea bag has tannic acid. This relives the infection and aids to get rid of the pain.

Honey

Honey has wonderful anti-bacterial properties. After brushing, put some amount of honey on the affected area of the gums. It works wonderfully to get rid of the gum infection.

Additional Tips

- Combine equal amounts of spinach juice and carrot juice and drink it once daily to maintain oral health.
- Increase intake of foods rich in vitamin C.
- Take a vitamin D supplement, after consulting a doctor, to improve oral health.
- Avoid food products made from refined sugar or refined grains.
- Munch on crunchy fruits and vegetables like guava, apples, radishes or cucumbers after your meals.
- Instead of using toothpicks, use dental floss to clean spaces between the teeth.
- Never go to bed without brushing your teeth at night.
- Have a good gargle after each meal to remove the food particles stuck between your teeth.
- Make sure to get regular dental checkups.

Conclusion

These are a few of the remedies that can help to prevent gum diseases or gives relief from the pain caused by bacterial gum infection. It is recommended that consulting a dentist in case of the problem prolongs for an period of time.

References

1. The American Academy of Periodontology. Proceedings of the World Workshop in Clinical Periodontics. Chicago: The American Academy of Periodontology, 1989, 23-24.

2. Ammons WF, Schectman LR, Page RC. Host tissue response in chronic periodontal disease. 1. The normal periodontium and clinical manifestations of dental and periodontal disease in the marmoset. Journal of periodontal research. 1972; 7(2):131-43. Doi:10.1111/j.1600-0765.1972.tb00638.x. PMID 4272039.

3. Page RC, Schroeder HE. Pathogenesis of inflammatory periodontal disease. A summary of current work. Laboratory Investigation. 1976; 34(3):235-49. PMID 765622.

4. Parameter on Plaque-Induced Gingivitis. Journal of Periodontology. 2000; 71(5):851-2. Doi: 10.1902/jop.2000.71.5-S.851. PMID 10875689.

5. Saini Rajiv, Saini Santosh, Saini Sugandha R. (2010-01-01). Periodontitis: A risk for delivery of premature labor and low-birth-weight infants. Journal of Natural Science, Biology, and Medicine. 1(1):40-42. Doi: 10.4103/0976-9668.71672. ISSN 0976-9668. PMC 3217279. PMID 22096335.

6. Research, Science and Therapy Committee of the American Academy of Periodontology. Treatment of Plaque-Induced Gingivitis, Chronic Periodontitis, and Other Clinical Conditions. Journal of Periodontology. 2001; 72(12):1790-1800. Doi: 10.1902/jop.2001.72.12.1790. PMID 11811516.

7. Kistler James O, Booth Veronica, Bradshaw David J, Wade William G, Glogauer Michael. (14 August). Bacterial Community Development in Experimental Gingivitis. PLoS ONE. 2013; 8(8):e71227. Doi: 10.1371/journal.pone.0071227.

8. Armitage Gary C. Development of a Classification System for Periodontal Diseases and Conditions (PDF). Annals of Periodontology. 4 (1):1-6. Doi:10.1902/annals.1999.4.1.1. PMID 10863 370. Archived from the original (PDF) on 2010-06-12.

9. Sambunjak D, Nickerson JW, Poklepovic T, Johnson TM, Imai P

Tugwell P *et al.* Johnson, Trevor M, ed. "Flossing for the management of periodontal diseases and dental caries in adults. The Cochrane Library. 2011; 12:CD008829. Doi: 10.1002/14651858.CD008829. Pub 2. PMID 22161438.

10. Hasturk AB, Hatice Nunn, Martha Warbington, Martha Van Dyke, Thomas E. Efficacy of a Fluoridated Hydrogen Peroxide-Based Mouthrinse for the Treatment of Gingivitis: A Randomized Clinical Trial. Journal of Periodontology. 2004; 75(1):57-65. Doi: 10.1902/jop. 2004.75.1.57. PMID15025217.

11. Deacon Scott A, Glenny Anne-Marie, Deery Chris, Robinson Peter G, Heanue Mike, Walmsley Damien A. Shaw William C (2010-12-08). Cochrane Database of Systematic Reviews. John Wiley & Sons, Ltd. doi: 10.1002/14651858.cd004971.pub2. PMID21154357.

12. American Dental Hygienists, Association Position Paper on the Oral Prophylaxis Archived 2012-06-26 at the Way back Machine, Approved by the ADHA Board of Trustees April 29, 1998.

13. FDA Triclosan: What Consumers Should Know Accessed, 2010, 08-12.

14. Yaacob M, Worthington HV, Deacon SA, Deery C, Walmsley AD, Robinson PG *et al.* (17 June). Powered versus manual toothbrushing for oral health. The Cochrane Database of Systematic Reviews, 2014, 6:CD00-2281. Doi: 10.1002/14651858.CD002281.pub3.PMID 2493438 3.

15. Stoeken Judith E, Paraskevas Spiros, Van Der Weijden, Godefridus A. The Long-Term Effect of a Mouthrinse Containing Essential Oils on Dental Plaque and Gingivitis: A Systematic Review. Journal of Periodontology. 2007; 78(7):1218-28. Doi: 10.1902/jop.2007.060269. PMID 17608576.